PCOS Diet Cookbook for Weight Loss

Nutrient-Rich Meals for Hormonal Balance
and Effective Weight Management

McDonnell B. Young

Copyright © 2024 by **McDonnell B. Young**
All rights reserved

No part of this publication may be reproduced, stored in a retrieval system, or transmitted, in any form or by any means, electronic, mechanical, photocopying, recording, or otherwise, without the prior written permission of the author.

The information in this ebook is true and complete to the best of our knowledge. All recommendation are made without guarantee on the part of author or publisher. The author and publisher disclaim any liability in connection with the use of this information.

Table of Contents

Introduction ... 5
   Understanding PCOS and Its Impact on Weight ... 8
   The Importance of Diet in Managing PCOS ... 11
   How to Use This Cookbook ... 14

Chapter 1: Breakfast Recipes ... 17
   Greek Yogurt with Berries and Chia Seeds ... 17
   Avocado and Egg Breakfast Sandwich ... 20
   Quinoa Breakfast Bowl with Nuts and Fruits ... 22
   Smoothie with Spinach, Banana, and Almond Butter ... 25
   Oatmeal with Flaxseeds and Blueberries ... 27
   Tofu Scramble with Veggies ... 29
   Cottage Cheese with Pineapple and Walnuts ... 32
   Whole Grain Toast with Mashed Avocado and Tomato ... 34
   Chia Pudding with Coconut Milk and Raspberries ... 36
   Egg Muffins with Spinach and Feta ... 38

Chapter 2: Lunch Recipes ... 40
   Grilled Chicken Salad with Avocado and Quinoa ... 40
   Lentil Soup with Spinach and Carrots ... 43
   Turkey and Hummus Wrap with Veggies ... 45
   Chickpea and Veggie Buddha Bowl ... 47
   Quinoa and Black Bean Salad with Cilantro Dressing ... 50
   Tuna Salad with Greek Yogurt and Dill ... 53
   Zucchini Noodles with Pesto and Cherry Tomatoes ... 55

Baked Salmon with Asparagus and Brown Rice	57
Veggie Stir-Fry with Tofu and Brown Rice	59
Stuffed Bell Peppers with Ground Turkey and Quinoa	62

Chapter 3: Dinner Recipes — 65

Baked Chicken Breast with Sweet Potato and Broccoli	65
Cauliflower Rice Stir-Fry with Shrimp	68
Grilled Steak with Green Beans and Quinoa	71
Spaghetti Squash with Turkey Meatballs	74
Baked Cod with Lemon and Asparagus	77
Stuffed Portobello Mushrooms with Spinach and Cheese	79
Beef and Veggie Skewers with Brown Rice	82
Eggplant Lasagna with Ricotta and Spinach	85
Herb-Crusted Pork Tenderloin with Roasted Vegetables	88
Chickpea Curry with Brown Rice and Spinach	91

Chapter 4: Snacks and Desserts — 94

Dark Chocolate and Almond Energy Bites	94
Greek Yogurt Parfait with Honey and Nuts	96
Chia Seed Pudding with Mango	99
Apple Slices with Almond Butter	101
Roasted Chickpeas with Spices	103

Conclusion — 105

Introduction

Once upon a sunny spring morning in the suburban town of Greenfield, Emily, a nutritionist with a vibrant practice, encountered her long-time client, Sarah. Sarah had been struggling with Polycystic Ovary Syndrome (PCOS) and weight gain, common woes that often brought clients to Emily's doorstep. Despite trying various diets and supplements, Sarah felt defeated by her minimal progress.

That day, Emily decided to introduce Sarah to her newly authored book, The PCOS Diet Cookbook for Weight Loss. As they sat in Emily's cozy office, sun filtering through the blinds, Emily handed her a beautifully bound copy. "This isn't just a cookbook," Emily explained, "it's a guide crafted specifically for those dealing with the unique challenges of PCOS."

The book was structured to educate and empower. The first section detailed how PCOS affects the body, emphasizing the importance of understanding insulin resistance, inflammation, and hormonal imbalance—all factors contributing to weight challenges. Emily had translated complex medical jargon into accessible, engaging language, accompanied by inspiring testimonials from women who had turned their lives around.

The core of the book was the meticulously curated recipes. Each recipe was designed not only to be delicious but also to stabilize insulin levels, reduce inflammation, and promote weight loss. Ingredients were easy to find, with a focus on whole foods known to benefit hormonal health, such as leafy greens, nuts, seeds, and lean proteins.

What set this cookbook apart was its practicality. Meal plans spanned all meals and snacks, crafted to fit busy lifestyles. The guide also offered modifications for vegans, vegetarians, and those with common food allergies, ensuring it was a versatile tool in any kitchen.

As Sarah flipped through the pages, she was drawn to the colorful photographs and the promise of simple, 30-minute recipes. There was even a section on understanding food labels and making smart grocery choices.

Emily pointed out another unique feature: a tracking journal. "Tracking your meals, symptoms, and progress can be incredibly empowering," she noted. "It helps you see the tangible benefits of dietary changes and motivates you to continue."

Sarah was sold. She felt that this guide was different—it was personalized, thoughtful, and comprehensive. The testimonials were relatable, and the scientific explanations helped her understand her body better. She could see herself using the meal plans and enjoying the food, a stark contrast to previous restrictive diets that left her feeling deprived.

Over the next few months, Sarah followed the book's guidance. The changes were gradual but noticeable. Not only did she start losing weight, but her energy levels improved, her skin cleared up, and even her mood swings diminished. The meals were satisfying, and she never felt like she was on a "diet."

At a follow-up appointment, Sarah excitedly shared her progress with Emily. She had lost 15 pounds, but more importantly, she felt in control of her health. "This book changed the way I see food and my condition," Sarah said, her eyes bright with gratitude.

Emily smiled, knowing she had made a difference. She hoped that The PCOS Diet Cookbook for Weight Loss would continue to reach more women like Sarah, helping them reclaim their health and vitality through the power of nourishing, balanced eating.

As Sarah left, cookbook in hand and a new optimism in her step, Emily felt a deep sense of fulfillment. This was why she had become a nutritionist—to make a tangible difference in people's lives, one meal at a time. And with her book, she was doing just that, far beyond the walls of her practice in Greenfield.

Understanding PCOS and Its Impact on Weight

Polycystic Ovary Syndrome (PCOS) is a complex hormonal disorder that affects approximately one in ten women of reproductive age, leading to various metabolic and hormonal imbalances. One of the most common symptoms of PCOS is weight gain or difficulty losing weight, largely due to the body's inability to use insulin effectively—a condition known as insulin resistance. This resistance prompts the pancreas to produce more insulin, which can increase fat storage in the body and make weight management challenging.

Women with PCOS often experience a cycle of weight gain that exacerbates other symptoms of the condition, such as irregular menstrual cycles, acne, hirsutism, and fertility issues. The relationship between PCOS and weight is bidirectional; excess weight can increase insulin levels, which worsens PCOS symptoms, creating a frustrating cycle of symptoms that can be difficult to break. Managing weight through dietary choices becomes a crucial aspect of managing PCOS overall.

The PCOS Diet Cookbook for Weight Loss addresses these challenges by focusing on foods that can help manage insulin levels and reduce inflammation. The recipes in the cookbook are rich in nutrients that balance hormones and improve metabolic health. Foods with a low glycemic index are emphasized because they cause a slower rise in blood glucose levels, which can help manage insulin resistance. This includes whole grains, legumes, nuts, seeds, and most vegetables and fruits, which are staples in the diet plan presented in the cookbook.

Beyond just managing insulin resistance, the cookbook also highlights the importance of incorporating anti-inflammatory foods into the diet. Chronic inflammation is a key player in PCOS, and a diet high in anti-inflammatory foods like berries, fatty fish, leafy greens, and olive oil can help reduce this inflammation. These dietary adjustments not only support weight loss but also contribute to overall hormonal balance, which can alleviate some of the symptoms associated with PCOS.

Moreover, the cookbook promotes a holistic approach to weight loss, emphasizing that diet should be enjoyable, sustainable, and adaptable to a woman's individual lifestyle. The recipes are designed to be simple and quick, recognizing that time constraints often present a significant barrier to preparing healthy meals. Each recipe includes modifications for different dietary needs, such as vegetarian or gluten-free options, ensuring that everyone can use this guide effectively.

The inclusion of a tracking journal within the cookbook serves as a tool for women to monitor their food intake, symptoms, and progress. This self-monitoring can enhance adherence to dietary changes by providing tangible feedback on how dietary choices influence symptoms and weight. It's a strategy that fosters a deeper connection to one's body and the impacts of nutrition on health.

By integrating tailored nutritional strategies with practical advice and supportive tools, The PCOS Diet Cookbook for Weight Loss empowers women to take control of their PCOS symptoms and improve their quality of life through sustainable weight management. This guide does more than just offer recipes; it offers a pathway to better health for countless women struggling with the effects of PCOS on their bodies and their lives.

The Importance of Diet in Managing PCOS

Polycystic Ovary Syndrome (PCOS) is a complex endocrine disorder that affects an estimated one in ten women of reproductive age. This condition is characterized by hormonal imbalances that can impact overall health and manifest in various symptoms, including weight gain, insulin resistance, irregular menstrual cycles, and infertility. Managing these symptoms often relies heavily on dietary changes, which can be both a preventative measure and a therapeutic approach. A specialized diet can help manage insulin levels and reduce inflammation, both of which are crucial in managing PCOS effectively.

The link between diet and the management of PCOS symptoms is rooted in the understanding of how certain foods influence the body's hormonal balance. Foods high in refined carbohydrates and sugars can exacerbate insulin resistance, a common issue in PCOS sufferers. Insulin resistance can lead to higher levels of insulin in the blood, which can increase the production of androgens and may worsen symptoms such as hirsutism, acne, and weight gain. Conversely, a diet rich in fiber, lean proteins, and anti-inflammatory foods can help stabilize blood sugar levels and reduce the impact of PCOS.

In relation to weight management, the role of diet becomes even more critical. Many women with PCOS experience difficulty losing weight due to insulin resistance and hormonal disruptions that influence metabolism. Adopting a diet that focuses on nutrient-dense, low-glycemic index foods can aid in weight loss by improving the body's use of insulin and decreasing appetite. The reduction in body weight can also help lower androgen levels and restore ovulation and regular menstrual cycles, thereby improving fertility in many cases.

The PCOS Diet Cookbook for Weight Loss addresses these dietary challenges directly, offering recipes and meal plans that cater to the needs of women struggling with PCOS. The cookbook emphasizes foods that contribute to a balanced, healthy diet, which can improve PCOS symptoms and support weight loss. It features meals that incorporate a variety of whole grains, lean proteins, and vegetables, all of which play a role in reducing insulin spikes and inflammation.

Moreover, the cookbook provides a practical approach to cooking and eating that does not require significant lifestyle changes, which can often be a barrier to maintaining a healthy diet. The recipes are designed to be simple, quick, and satisfying, making it easier for individuals with busy lives to stick to a healthful eating plan. This ease of use encourages consistency, which is key in managing a chronic condition like PCOS.

Another benefit of the cookbook is its attention to the emotional and psychological aspects of dealing with PCOS. It encourages a positive relationship with food, which is essential as many women with PCOS may struggle with body image issues due to weight gain and other visible symptoms of the disorder. By promoting a healthy attitude towards food and eating, the cookbook supports not only physical health but also mental and emotional well-being.

In conclusion, managing PCOS with a targeted diet is not just about weight loss but about creating a sustainable, healthy lifestyle that addresses the underlying causes of PCOS symptoms. The PCOS Diet Cookbook for Weight Loss serves as an invaluable resource for women to take control of their health through informed dietary choices. It stands as a testament to the power of food as medicine and the importance of dietary management in overcoming the challenges of PCOS.

How to Use This Cookbook

In crafting a user-friendly approach, this cookbook is structured to assist individuals managing PCOS in navigating their dietary needs efficiently while aiming for weight loss. It begins by explaining the function of each recipe, linking it with how the ingredients can positively influence PCOS symptoms and weight management. Each recipe is flagged for its specific benefits, like anti-inflammatory properties or insulin regulation, which educates readers on why certain foods are chosen and how they can alter their diet according to specific symptoms they may experience.

To simplify meal preparation, the recipes are designed with practicality in mind, suitable for both novice cooks and seasoned kitchen enthusiasts. Every recipe requires minimal, readily available ingredients and straightforward steps to avoid any kitchen hassle. The aim is to reduce time spent in the kitchen while maximizing nutritional benefits, ensuring meals can be prepared within 30 minutes or less. This practicality supports consistent adherence to the diet, making it easier to maintain over time.

Portion control is a critical aspect highlighted throughout the book, tailored to meet calorie intake that complements a

PCOS-friendly diet for weight loss. Each recipe provides detailed nutritional information, including calorie counts, macronutrient breakdown, and serving size suggestions. This detailed guidance helps readers understand how to fit each meal into their daily caloric needs without the guesswork.

Adaptability of the recipes to various dietary restrictions plays a significant role in the cookbook's layout. Variations for vegan, gluten-free, or dairy-free diets are provided, ensuring that the recipes are inclusive. These adaptations are not afterthoughts but are integrated into the recipe's core instructions, offering substitutions that maintain the flavor and nutritional value of the meals, ensuring everyone, regardless of dietary restrictions, can benefit.

Meal planning is made seamless with the inclusion of weekly meal planner templates that consider the comprehensive needs of a PCOS diet. These planners help in organizing meals for the week, incorporating a balanced mix of carbohydrates, proteins, and fats, along with necessary fiber and micronutrients to manage PCOS effectively. The templates also help in grocery shopping, as they are designed to utilize ingredients across multiple recipes to minimize waste and cost.

Beyond the kitchen, the cookbook encourages a holistic approach to managing PCOS through additional lifestyle tips that complement the dietary advice. Stress management techniques, importance of regular physical activity, and tips for consistent sleep schedules are discussed, providing a well-rounded guide to managing PCOS symptoms holistically.

Finally, the cookbook fosters a supportive community through encouragement to share experiences and recipes. It invites readers to engage with each other online, sharing successes and challenges, fostering a sense of community and support among individuals with PCOS. This aspect of community building not only motivates continued adherence to the dietary guidelines but also enhances the overall journey towards health and wellness with PCOS, making the path to weight loss more achievable and less isolating.

Chapter 1: Breakfast Recipes

Greek Yogurt with Berries and Chia Seeds

Ingredients:

- 1 cup plain Greek yogurt (low-fat or full-fat depending on dietary preference)
- 1/2 cup mixed berries (such as blueberries, strawberries, and raspberries), fresh or frozen
- 1 tablespoon chia seeds
- Optional: a drizzle of honey or pure maple syrup for added sweetness

Instructions:

1. In a serving bowl, place the Greek yogurt.
2. Top the yogurt with the mixed berries. If using frozen berries, allow them to thaw slightly at room temperature for a juicier blend.
3. Sprinkle the chia seeds evenly over the berries.
4. If a touch of sweetness is desired, drizzle honey or maple syrup over the top.

5. Stir the mixture slightly to combine the flavors and allow to sit for 5 minutes. This resting time lets the chia seeds swell slightly, adding a pleasant texture.

Nutritional Information:

- Calories: Approximately 290 kcal per serving
- Protein: 20g
- Fat: 9g (with minimal saturated fat, depending on the type of Greek yogurt used)
- Carbohydrates: 33g
- Fiber: 5g
- Sugars: 18g (natural sugars from the berries and optional honey/maple syrup)

Serving Size: This recipe serves 1, making it easy to prepare and perfect for a quick morning meal.

Cooking Time: The total preparation time is about 5 minutes, making it an ideal choice for those busy mornings when time is scarce but nourishment is needed.

Avocado and Egg Breakfast Sandwich

Ingredients:

- 1 ripe avocado
- 2 eggs
- 2 whole grain English muffins
- 1 tablespoon olive oil
- Salt and pepper to taste
- Optional: slices of tomato or leafy greens like spinach or arugula

Instructions:

1. Heat a non-stick skillet over medium heat and add olive oil.
2. Crack the eggs into the pan and cook to your preference, either scrambled or fried.
3. While the eggs are cooking, slice the avocado and season it with salt and pepper.
4. Toast the English muffins until they are golden brown.
5. Assemble the sandwich by layering the sliced avocado on the bottom half of each muffin, followed by the cooked egg. If using, add tomato slices or greens.
6. Cap with the top half of the muffin and serve warm.

Nutritional Information:

Each serving of the Avocado and Egg Breakfast Sandwich provides approximately:

- Calories: 400
- Protein: 17g
- Fat: 23g (primarily monounsaturated fat)
- Carbohydrates: 33g
- Fiber: 9g

Serving Size:

This recipe serves 2, with each serving consisting of one sandwich.

Cooking Time:

Preparation and cooking time is about 15 minutes, making it a quick and nutritious choice to start the day.

Quinoa Breakfast Bowl with Nuts and Fruits

Ingredients:

- 1 cup cooked quinoa
- 1/4 cup sliced almonds
- 1/4 cup chopped walnuts
- 1/2 cup fresh blueberries
- 1/2 cup sliced strawberries
- 1 tablespoon chia seeds
- 1 teaspoon cinnamon
- Honey or maple syrup (optional, to taste)
- 1 cup unsweetened almond milk

Instructions:

1. Prepare the quinoa according to package instructions. Allow it to cool slightly.
2. In a serving bowl, combine the cooked quinoa with almond milk, stirring until well mixed.
3. Top the quinoa with sliced almonds, chopped walnuts, blueberries, and strawberries.
4. Sprinkle chia seeds and cinnamon over the top.

5. Drizzle a small amount of honey or maple syrup if a sweeter taste is desired.
6. Serve immediately for a fresh, warm breakfast, or refrigerate overnight for a chilled version.

Nutritional Information:

This breakfast is designed to provide a balanced blend of macronutrients vital for PCOS management. It offers approximately:
- Calories: 350
- Protein: 9 grams
- Fats: 15 grams (healthy fats from nuts and chia seeds)
- Carbohydrates: 50 grams (complex carbohydrates from quinoa and fruits)
- Fiber: 8 grams

Serving Size:

This recipe serves 1, making it easy to manage portion size for effective weight management.

Cooking Time:

The total time required to prepare the Quinoa Breakfast Bowl is about 20 minutes if starting with uncooked quinoa, or just 10 minutes if using precooked or leftover quinoa from a previous meal.

Smoothie with Spinach, Banana, and Almond Butter

Ingredients:

- 1 cup fresh spinach
- 1 ripe banana
- 2 tablespoons almond butter
- 1 cup unsweetened almond milk
- 1 tablespoon flaxseeds
- Ice cubes (optional for a thicker smoothie)

Instructions:

1. Place the spinach, peeled banana, almond butter, and flaxseeds into a blender.
2. Add the almond milk and a handful of ice cubes if a thicker consistency is preferred.
3. Blend on high until all the ingredients are completely smooth.
4. Pour into a glass and serve immediately for best taste and nutrient retention.

Nutritional Information:

- Calories: 325

- Protein: 8 grams
- Fat: 18 grams (including healthy fats from almond butter and flaxseeds)
- Carbohydrates: 36 grams
- Fiber: 7 grams
- Sugar: 14 grams

Serving Size: This recipe serves 1, making it a quick and easy breakfast option that doesn't require complicated measurements or scaling.

Cooking Time: The total time from preparation to serving is approximately 5 minutes, making it an ideal choice for busy mornings.

Oatmeal with Flaxseeds and Blueberries

Ingredients:

- 1 cup of rolled oats
- 2 cups of water or unsweetened almond milk
- 2 tablespoons of ground flaxseeds
- 1/2 cup of fresh blueberries
- 1 tablespoon of honey or pure maple syrup (optional)
- 1/4 teaspoon of cinnamon (optional)

Instructions:

1. In a small pot, bring the water or almond milk to a boil.
2. Add the rolled oats and simmer on low heat, stirring occasionally, until the oats are soft and have absorbed most of the liquid, about 5-7 minutes.
3. Remove the pot from heat and stir in the ground flaxseeds and cinnamon.
4. Cover the pot and let sit for a couple of minutes for the flaxseeds to soften.
5. Serve the oatmeal topped with fresh blueberries and a drizzle of honey or maple syrup if desired.

Nutritional Information:

- Calories: 350
- Protein: 9 grams
- Carbohydrates: 50 grams
- Fat: 12 grams (mainly from flaxseeds, which are high in healthy fats)
- Fiber: 8 grams

Serving Size:

- This recipe serves 1. It can be doubled or tripled to serve more, maintaining the ratio of oats to liquid.

Cooking Time:

- Total preparation and cooking time is approximately 10-12 minutes, making it a quick and efficient option for a healthy breakfast.

Tofu Scramble with Veggies

Ingredients:

- 1 tablespoon olive oil
- 1/2 block firm tofu, crumbled
- 1/2 teaspoon turmeric
- 1/4 teaspoon black salt (for an eggy flavor)
- 1 red bell pepper, diced
- 1 small zucchini, diced
- 1/2 cup chopped spinach
- 1/4 cup cherry tomatoes, halved
- Salt and pepper, to taste
- 1/4 teaspoon paprika
- Fresh herbs (like parsley or cilantro) for garnish

Instructions:

1. Heat olive oil in a non-stick skillet over medium heat.
2. Add crumbled tofu and turmeric, stirring until the tofu is evenly coated. Cook for about 5 minutes until the tofu starts to get slightly golden.
3. Sprinkle black salt over the tofu for an eggy flavor.

4. Add the diced red bell pepper and zucchini to the skillet, cooking for an additional 5-7 minutes until the vegetables are tender.
5. Stir in the chopped spinach and cherry tomatoes, cooking for another 2-3 minutes until the spinach wilts and tomatoes are just warm.
6. Season with salt, pepper, and paprika, adjusting to taste.
7. Remove from heat and garnish with fresh herbs before serving.

Nutritional Information:

- Calories: 250
- Protein: 18g
- Carbohydrates: 15g
- Fat: 14g
- Fiber: 5g
- Sugar: 6g

Serving Size:

This recipe serves 2. Each serving is a generous and fulfilling plate that provides a balanced mix of protein, fats, and carbohydrates.

Cooking Time:

Preparation and cooking time is approximately 20 minutes, making it a quick and efficient option for a busy morning.

Cottage Cheese with Pineapple and Walnuts

Ingredients:

- 1 cup low-fat cottage cheese
- 1/2 cup chopped fresh pineapple
- 1/4 cup walnuts, roughly chopped
- Optional: a drizzle of honey or a sprinkle of cinnamon for added flavor

Instructions:

1. In a serving bowl, place the cottage cheese.
2. Top the cottage cheese with the freshly chopped pineapple and walnuts.
3. For an added touch of sweetness or spice, drizzle a little honey over the top or sprinkle some cinnamon.
4. Mix gently to combine the ingredients just before eating to enjoy the blend of textures and flavors.

Nutritional Information:

- Calories: 345
- Protein: 20g

- Carbohydrates: 20g
- Fat: 20g
- Sugars: 15g
- Fiber: 2g

Serving Size: This recipe serves one, making it easy to manage portions and nutritional intake, which is crucial for weight loss and managing PCOS symptoms.

Cooking Time: The preparation time is about 5 minutes, as there is no cooking involved, making it a quick and easy option for a busy morning.

Whole Grain Toast with Mashed Avocado and Tomato

Ingredients:

- 2 slices of whole grain bread
- 1 ripe avocado
- 1 small tomato, sliced
- Salt and pepper to taste
- Optional: a sprinkle of crushed red pepper flakes or fresh herbs like basil or parsley for garnish

Instructions:

1. Toast the whole grain bread slices to your preferred crispness.
2. While the bread is toasting, peel and pit the avocado. In a small bowl, mash the avocado with a fork until it reaches a smooth consistency.
3. Spread the mashed avocado evenly over the toasted bread.
4. Arrange the tomato slices over the mashed avocado.
5. Season with salt and pepper to taste, and if desired, add red pepper flakes or fresh herbs for extra flavor.
6. Serve immediately to enjoy the freshness of the ingredients.

Nutritional Information:

This meal is high in fiber, which helps in managing insulin levels—a crucial element in PCOS management. Avocados provide heart-healthy monounsaturated fats and nearly 20 different vitamins and minerals, making them a great food for hormonal balance and inflammation reduction. Tomatoes add vitamin C, potassium, folate, and vitamin K.

Serving Size:

- Serves 1 person. Each serving includes 2 slices of whole grain toast topped with avocado and tomato.

Cooking Time:

- Prep time: 5 minutes
- Cook time: 2 minutes (for toasting the bread)
- Total time: 7 minutes

Chia Pudding with Coconut Milk and Raspberries

Ingredients:

- 1/4 cup chia seeds
- 1 cup unsweetened coconut milk
- 1/2 teaspoon vanilla extract
- 1 tablespoon honey or maple syrup (optional)
- 1/2 cup fresh raspberries
- A pinch of salt

Instructions:

1. In a medium bowl, mix the chia seeds and coconut milk together. Add the vanilla extract and a pinch of salt. Stir in honey or maple syrup if a sweeter taste is desired.
2. Cover the bowl and refrigerate overnight or for at least 6 hours until the mixture achieves a pudding-like consistency.
3. Once set, stir the pudding to check consistency. If it's too thick, add a bit more coconut milk to loosen it.
4. Serve the pudding in bowls or glasses and top with fresh raspberries.

Nutritional Information:

Each serving of this chia pudding provides approximately:
- Calories: 215
- Carbohydrates: 20g
- Fiber: 10g
- Protein: 4g
- Fat: 14g

Serving Size:

This recipe yields two servings, making it ideal for a filling single breakfast or to share for a lighter start.

Cooking Time:

The preparation time is about 5 minutes, although the pudding must be refrigerated overnight or for at least 6 hours to set properly. This make-ahead nature ensures a quick and easy breakfast option, perfect for busy mornings.

Egg Muffins with Spinach and Feta

Ingredients:

- 6 large eggs
- 1 cup fresh spinach, chopped
- 1/2 cup feta cheese, crumbled
- 1/4 cup onions, finely chopped
- 1/4 cup red bell peppers, diced
- Salt and pepper to taste
- Cooking spray or a dab of olive oil for greasing

Instructions:

1. Preheat the oven to 375 degrees Fahrenheit (190 degrees Celsius).
2. Grease a muffin tin with cooking spray or olive oil.
3. In a bowl, whisk the eggs until well beaten. Stir in the chopped spinach, feta cheese, onions, and bell peppers. Season with salt and pepper.
4. Pour the egg mixture evenly into the muffin tins, filling each cup about two-thirds full.
5. Bake in the preheated oven for 20-25 minutes, or until the tops are firm to the touch and eggs are cooked through.

6. Allow to cool for a few minutes before removing from the tin. Serve warm.

Nutritional Information:

Each muffin contains approximately:

- Calories: 100
- Protein: 7 grams
- Fat: 7 grams (with 3 grams of saturated fat from the feta)
- Carbohydrates: 2 grams
- Fiber: 0.5 grams
- Sugar: 1 gram

Serving Size:

This recipe makes 12 muffins. A single serving is typically 2 muffins, making it sufficient to start the day feeling full and energized.

Cooking Time:

Preparation time is about 10 minutes, with an additional 20-25 minutes for baking. This makes the total time from start to finish approximately 30-35 minutes.

Chapter 2: Lunch Recipes

Grilled Chicken Salad with Avocado and Quinoa

Ingredients:

- 2 boneless, skinless chicken breasts
- 1 tablespoon olive oil
- Salt and pepper, to taste
- 1 cup cooked quinoa
- 1 avocado, sliced
- 2 cups mixed greens (like arugula and spinach)
- 1/2 cucumber, sliced
- 1/4 red onion, thinly sliced
- 2 tablespoons chopped fresh cilantro
- Juice of 1 lime
- 2 tablespoons extra virgin olive oil
- 1 teaspoon honey (optional)

Instructions:

1. Preheat the grill to medium-high heat. Rub the chicken breasts with olive oil and season with salt and pepper.

2. Grill the chicken for 6-7 minutes per side, or until fully cooked and the internal temperature reaches 165°F. Let it rest for a few minutes and then slice thinly.
3. In a large bowl, combine the mixed greens, cooked quinoa, cucumber, red onion, and cilantro.
4. In a small bowl, whisk together the lime juice, extra virgin olive oil, and honey if using, to make the dressing.
5. Add the sliced chicken and avocado to the salad, drizzle with the dressing, and toss everything together to combine.
6. Serve immediately.

Nutritional Information:

- Calories: 350 per serving
- Protein: 26g
- Carbohydrates: 27g
- Fat: 16g
- Fiber: 6g

Serving Size:

This recipe serves 2.

Cooking Time:

Total preparation and cooking time is approximately 20 minutes.

Lentil Soup with Spinach and Carrots

Ingredients:

- 1 cup dried lentils, rinsed
- 1 large carrot, diced
- 2 cups spinach leaves, roughly chopped
- 1 onion, finely chopped
- 2 cloves garlic, minced
- 1 teaspoon ground cumin
- 1/2 teaspoon ground coriander
- 4 cups vegetable broth
- 2 tablespoons olive oil
- Salt and pepper to taste
- 1 tablespoon lemon juice (optional)

Instructions:

1. In a large pot, heat the olive oil over medium heat. Add the onion and garlic, sautéing until the onion becomes translucent.
2. Stir in the carrots and cook for about 3 minutes until slightly softened.
3. Add the lentils, cumin, and coriander, mixing well to combine with the vegetables.

4. Pour in the vegetable broth and bring the mixture to a boil. Once boiling, reduce the heat and let simmer uncovered for about 20 minutes, or until the lentils are tender.
5. Add the chopped spinach to the pot and continue to simmer for another 5 minutes. Season with salt and pepper to taste.
6. Remove from heat and stir in lemon juice if using. Serve hot.

Nutritional Information:

Each serving of this soup is rich in dietary fiber, protein, and essential nutrients like iron and magnesium, which are vital for managing insulin levels and supporting metabolic health. The soup is low in calories, with each serving containing approximately 220 calories, 14 grams of protein, and 35 grams of carbohydrates.

Serving Size:

This recipe serves 4 people. It's perfect for a fulfilling lunch that doesn't leave you feeling weighed down.

Cooking Time:

Total preparation and cooking time is approximately 35 minutes, making this an excellent choice for a quick, nutritious midday meal.

Turkey and Hummus Wrap with Veggies

Ingredients:

- 1 whole wheat tortilla (8-inch diameter)
- 3 ounces of thinly sliced turkey breast
- 2 tablespoons of hummus
- 1/4 cup of shredded carrots
- 1/4 cup of sliced cucumber
- 1/4 cup of red bell pepper strips
- 1/4 cup of baby spinach leaves
- 1 teaspoon of olive oil
- 1 tablespoon of lemon juice
- Salt and pepper to taste

Instructions:

1. Start by laying the whole wheat tortilla flat on a clean surface.
2. Spread the hummus evenly over the surface of the tortilla.
3. Arrange the turkey slices across the center of the tortilla on top of the hummus.
4. Toss the shredded carrots, sliced cucumber, and red bell pepper strips in olive oil, lemon juice, and a pinch of salt and pepper.

5. Add the vegetable mixture over the turkey slices, and top with baby spinach leaves.

6. Carefully roll the tortilla, folding in the edges to hold the fillings.

7. Cut the wrap in half diagonally and serve immediately or wrap it up for a grab-and-go lunch.

Nutritional Information:

- Calories: 330
- Carbohydrates: 35g
- Protein: 25g
- Fat: 12g
- Fiber: 6g
- Sugar: 3g

Serving Size:

- This recipe serves 1, making it easy to manage portions and keep track of nutritional intake.

Cooking Time:

- Preparation time: 10 minutes
- No cooking required

Chickpea and Veggie Buddha Bowl

Ingredients:

- 1 cup cooked chickpeas, drained and rinsed
- 1 small sweet potato, peeled and cubed
- 1 cup kale, washed and chopped
- 1/2 cup red cabbage, shredded
- 1 medium carrot, julienned
- 1/4 cup red onion, thinly sliced
- 1 tablespoon olive oil
- Salt and pepper, to taste
- 2 tablespoons tahini
- 1 tablespoon lemon juice
- 1 garlic clove, minced
- 1/4 teaspoon paprika
- Water (as needed for dressing consistency)

Instructions:

1. Preheat the oven to 400°F (200°C).
2. Toss the sweet potato cubes with half the olive oil, salt, and pepper, and spread them out on a baking sheet. Roast in the oven for 25-30 minutes until tender and lightly browned.

3. In a large bowl, combine the roasted sweet potatoes, chickpeas, kale, red cabbage, carrot, and red onion.

4. In a small bowl, whisk together the tahini, remaining olive oil, lemon juice, minced garlic, paprika, and water as needed to achieve a dressing-like consistency. Season with salt and pepper to taste.

5. Drizzle the dressing over the salad and toss everything together until well coated.

Nutritional Information:

- Calories: 350
- Protein: 12 grams
- Fat: 14 grams (primarily from olive oil and tahini, which are good sources of healthy fats)
- Carbohydrates: 45 grams
- Fiber: 11 grams

Serving Size:

This recipe serves 2, making it easy to adjust for a single serving or for a family meal by simply doubling the ingredients.

Cooking Time:

Preparation takes around 15 minutes, and cooking time is approximately 30 minutes, making the total time from start to finish about 45 minutes.

Quinoa and Black Bean Salad with Cilantro Dressing

Ingredients:

- 1 cup quinoa
- 2 cups water
- 1 can (15 ounces) black beans, drained and rinsed
- 1 medium red bell pepper, diced
- 1 medium cucumber, diced
- 1/4 cup finely chopped red onion
- 1/4 cup chopped fresh cilantro
- Salt and pepper to taste
- 1/4 cup extra virgin olive oil
- Juice of 1 lime
- 1 clove garlic, minced
- 1/4 cup fresh cilantro, finely chopped
- Salt and pepper to taste

Instructions:

1. Rinse the quinoa under cold running water until the water runs clear. Combine the rinsed quinoa and water in a medium saucepan and bring to a boil over high heat. Reduce heat to low,

cover, and simmer until the quinoa is tender and the water has been absorbed, about 15 minutes. Remove from heat and let stand, covered, for 5 minutes. Fluff with a fork and allow to cool slightly.
2. In a large bowl, combine the cooled quinoa, black beans, red bell pepper, cucumber, and red onion.
3. In a small bowl, whisk together the olive oil, lime juice, minced garlic, and chopped cilantro for the dressing. Season with salt and pepper to taste.
4. Pour the dressing over the quinoa mixture and toss to combine. Adjust seasoning as needed.
5. Garnish with additional cilantro before serving.

Nutritional Information (per serving):

- Calories: 320
- Protein: 11 grams
- Fat: 10 grams
- Carbohydrates: 45 grams
- Fiber: 9 grams
- Sugar: 3 grams

Serving Size:

- Makes 4 servings.

Cooking Time:
- Total time from start to finish is about 30 minutes, with 15 minutes of cooking and 15 minutes of preparation time.

Tuna Salad with Greek Yogurt and Dill

Ingredients:

- 2 cans of tuna in water, drained
- 1 cup Greek yogurt, plain
- 2 tablespoons fresh dill, chopped
- 1/2 cup celery, finely chopped
- 1/4 cup red onion, finely chopped
- 1 tablespoon lemon juice
- Salt and pepper to taste
- Lettuce leaves or whole grain bread for serving

Instructions:

1. In a mixing bowl, combine the drained tuna, Greek yogurt, and lemon juice. Mix thoroughly to break up the tuna and integrate the yogurt smoothly.
2. Add the chopped dill, celery, and red onion to the tuna mixture. Stir until all ingredients are well combined.
3. Season the mixture with salt and pepper according to taste.
4. Chill the salad in the refrigerator for at least 30 minutes before serving to allow the flavors to meld together.

5. Serve the chilled tuna salad on a bed of crisp lettuce leaves or as a sandwich filling between slices of whole grain bread.

Nutritional Information:

- Calories: 180 per serving
- Protein: 22g
- Fat: 4g (1g saturated)
- Carbohydrates: 6g
- Fiber: 1g
- Sugar: 4g

Serving Size:

This recipe serves four, making it perfect for individual meal prep or a family lunch.

Cooking Time:

The preparation time is approximately 10 minutes, with an additional 30 minutes recommended for chilling.

Zucchini Noodles with Pesto and Cherry Tomatoes

Ingredients:

- 4 medium zucchinis, spiralized
- 1 cup cherry tomatoes, halved
- 1/2 cup fresh basil leaves
- 2 cloves garlic
- 1/4 cup pine nuts
- 1/3 cup extra virgin olive oil
- Salt and pepper, to taste
- Parmesan cheese, grated (optional for topping)

Instructions:

1. In a food processor, combine basil leaves, garlic, pine nuts, and a pinch of salt and pepper. Pulse until coarsely chopped.
2. Gradually pour in the olive oil while the processor is running until a smooth pesto forms.
3. In a large skillet, heat a small amount of olive oil over medium heat. Add the spiralized zucchini noodles and sauté for about 2-3 minutes, just until tender.

4. Remove the skillet from heat and mix in the pesto to evenly coat the noodles.
5. Gently toss the cherry tomatoes with the zucchini noodles.
6. Serve warm, topped with grated Parmesan if desired.

Nutritional Information:

Each serving of this recipe provides approximately:
- Calories: 250
- Carbohydrates: 10g
- Protein: 5g
- Fat: 22g
- Fiber: 3g
- Sugar: 5g

Serving Size:

This recipe serves 4, with each serving consisting of about 1 cup of zucchini noodles and a generous tablespoon of pesto.

Cooking Time:

The total preparation and cooking time for this meal is about 15 minutes, making it a quick and efficient option for a busy day.

Baked Salmon with Asparagus and Brown Rice

Ingredients:

- 4 salmon fillets (4-6 oz each)
- 1 bunch of asparagus, trimmed
- 1 cup brown rice
- 2 tablespoons olive oil
- Salt and pepper to taste
- Lemon wedges for garnish

Instructions:

1. Preheat the oven to 400 degrees Fahrenheit.
2. Rinse brown rice under cold water until water runs clear. Cook according to package instructions, typically about 45 minutes, until water is absorbed and rice is tender.
3. While the rice cooks, line a baking sheet with parchment paper. Place salmon fillets and asparagus on the sheet. Drizzle with olive oil and season with salt and pepper.
4. Bake in the preheated oven for 12-15 minutes, or until salmon is flaky and asparagus is tender-crisp.

5. Serve the baked salmon and asparagus over a bed of brown rice. Garnish with lemon wedges.

Nutritional Information:

- Calories: 480
- Protein: 34g
- Fat: 22g (Saturated Fat: 3g; Omega-3 Fatty Acids: 4g)
- Carbohydrates: 36g
- Fiber: 5g
- Sugar: 2g
- Sodium: 70mg

Serving Size: This recipe serves 4, with each serving including one salmon fillet, a quarter of the asparagus, and a 1/4 cup cooked brown rice.

Cooking Time: Total preparation and cooking time is approximately 60 minutes, which includes the simultaneous preparation of the rice and the baking of the salmon and asparagus.

Veggie Stir-Fry with Tofu and Brown Rice

Ingredients:

- 1 cup brown rice, uncooked
- 2 tablespoons olive oil
- 4 cups mixed vegetables (broccoli, bell peppers, carrots, and snap peas)
- 200 grams firm tofu, cubed
- 2 cloves garlic, minced
- 1 tablespoon ginger, grated
- 2 tablespoons soy sauce (or tamari for a gluten-free option)
- 1 tablespoon sesame oil
- Salt and pepper to taste
- Optional: sesame seeds and chopped green onions for garnish

Instructions:

1. Cook the brown rice according to package instructions. Typically, this involves bringing 2 cups of water to a boil, adding the rice, and letting it simmer covered for about 45 minutes until tender.

2. While the rice cooks, heat the olive oil in a large skillet or wok over medium-high heat. Add the garlic and ginger, sautéing for about 30 seconds until fragrant.
3. Increase the heat to high and add the mixed vegetables. Stir-fry for about 5 minutes until just tender but still crisp.
4. Add the tofu cubes to the skillet, tossing to combine. Cook for an additional 5 minutes, allowing the tofu to brown slightly.
5. Drizzle the soy sauce and sesame oil over the mixture, stirring well to coat all ingredients evenly. Season with salt and pepper.
6. Serve the stir-fry over the cooked brown rice, garnished with sesame seeds and green onions if desired.

Nutritional Information:

Each serving provides a balanced mix of carbohydrates, proteins, and fats. Specifically, one serving contains approximately:
- Calories: 350
- Carbohydrates: 45 g
- Protein: 15 g
- Fat: 15 g
- Fiber: 6 g
- Sugars: 5 g

Serving Size:

This recipe serves four, making it an excellent option for a family lunch or planned leftovers, which can simplify meal preparation for the week.

Cooking Time:

The total preparation and cooking time is about 60 minutes, with 45 minutes allocated for cooking the rice and 15 minutes for preparing and cooking the stir-fry.

Stuffed Bell Peppers with Ground Turkey and Quinoa

Ingredients:

- 4 large bell peppers, any color, tops cut off and seeded
- 1 tablespoon olive oil
- 1 medium onion, finely chopped
- 2 cloves garlic, minced
- 1 pound ground turkey
- 1 cup cooked quinoa
- 1 can (14.5 ounces) diced tomatoes, drained
- 1 teaspoon salt
- 1/2 teaspoon black pepper
- 2 teaspoons dried oregano
- 1/2 cup shredded mozzarella cheese (optional)

Instructions:

1. Preheat your oven to 375°F (190°C).
2. In a skillet over medium heat, heat the olive oil and sauté onion and garlic until they are soft, about 3-4 minutes.
3. Add the ground turkey to the skillet and cook until browned, breaking it up as it cooks, about 5-7 minutes.

4. Stir in the cooked quinoa, diced tomatoes, salt, pepper, and oregano. Cook together for another 5 minutes until everything is well combined.
5. Spoon the turkey and quinoa mixture into the hollowed-out bell peppers, and place them in a baking dish.
6. Cover with aluminum foil and bake in the preheated oven for 35 minutes.
7. Remove the foil, top each pepper with mozzarella cheese if using, and bake for another 10 minutes, or until the cheese is melted and bubbly.
8. Let the peppers stand for about 5 minutes before serving.

Nutritional Information:

Each stuffed pepper is a powerhouse of nutrients. It contains approximately:
- Calories: 320
- Protein: 26g
- Fat: 14g (with cheese) / 9g (without cheese)
- Carbohydrates: 28g
- Fiber: 5g
- Sugars: 8g

Serving Size:

This recipe serves four, with one stuffed pepper per serving. It is designed to be a complete meal on its own, providing enough energy and satisfaction without the need for side dishes.

Cooking Time:

The total cooking time for this recipe is about 55 minutes, with 15 minutes of preparation time and 40 minutes of cooking time, making it an excellent choice for a weekend meal prep or a comforting weeknight dinner.

Chapter 3: Dinner Recipes

Baked Chicken Breast with Sweet Potato and Broccoli

Ingredients:

- 4 boneless, skinless chicken breasts
- 2 large sweet potatoes, peeled and cubed
- 2 heads of broccoli, cut into florets
- 2 tablespoons olive oil
- 1 teaspoon garlic powder
- 1 teaspoon paprika
- Salt and pepper to taste

Instructions:

1. Preheat the oven to 400 degrees Fahrenheit (200 degrees Celsius).
2. In a large bowl, toss the sweet potato cubes and broccoli florets with olive oil, garlic powder, paprika, salt, and pepper until they are evenly coated.
3. Spread the vegetables on a baking sheet in a single layer, leaving space in the center for the chicken breasts.

4. Place the chicken breasts in the center of the baking sheet. Season them with salt, pepper, and additional paprika.

5. Place the baking sheet in the oven and bake for about 25-30 minutes, or until the chicken is thoroughly cooked and the vegetables are tender and slightly caramelized.

6. Remove from oven and let sit for a few minutes before serving to allow the juices to redistribute in the chicken.

Nutritional Information:

Each serving contains approximately:

- Calories: 310
- Protein: 30g
- Carbohydrates: 33g
- Fiber: 6g
- Fat: 8g
- Sugar: 7g

Serving Size:

This recipe serves 4. Each serving consists of one chicken breast, a half of a sweet potato, and a quarter of the broccoli florets.

Cooking Time:

Preparation time is around 10 minutes, with a cooking time of 25-30 minutes, totaling approximately 40 minutes from start to finish.

Cauliflower Rice Stir-Fry with Shrimp

Ingredients:

- 1 medium head of cauliflower, grated into rice-sized pieces
- 1 pound of shrimp, peeled and deveined
- 1 tablespoon of olive oil
- 1 red bell pepper, thinly sliced
- 1 cup of snap peas
- 2 cloves garlic, minced
- 1 teaspoon of ginger, minced
- 2 tablespoons of soy sauce (or tamari for a gluten-free option)
- 1 tablespoon of sesame oil
- 1/4 teaspoon of crushed red pepper flakes (optional)
- Salt and pepper to taste
- Fresh cilantro or green onions for garnish

Instructions:

1. Heat the olive oil in a large skillet over medium-high heat. Add the minced garlic and ginger, sautéing until fragrant, about 1 minute.

2. Add the shrimp to the skillet and cook until they turn pink and are cooked through, about 3-4 minutes per side. Remove the shrimp from the skillet and set aside.

3. In the same skillet, add a bit more olive oil if needed, and then the bell pepper and snap peas. Stir-fry for about 2-3 minutes until they start to soften.

4. Stir in the cauliflower rice, soy sauce, sesame oil, and red pepper flakes if using. Continue to stir-fry for about 5-7 minutes, or until the cauliflower is tender.

5. Return the shrimp to the skillet and stir everything together until well combined and heated through.

6. Season with salt and pepper to taste. Garnish with chopped cilantro or green onions before serving.

Nutritional Information (per serving):

- Calories: 250
- Fat: 10g
- Carbohydrates: 15g
- Fiber: 5g
- Protein: 25g
- Sugar: 5g

Serving Size: Serves 4

Cooking Time: Preparation takes about 10 minutes, and cooking time is approximately 15 minutes, making this dish quick and easy for a nutritious lunch.

Grilled Steak with Green Beans and Quinoa

Ingredients:

- 6 oz lean steak
- 1 cup fresh green beans, trimmed
- 1/2 cup quinoa
- 2 cloves garlic, minced
- 1 tablespoon olive oil
- Salt and pepper to taste
- Fresh herbs (like parsley or thyme) for garnish

Instructions:

1. Rinse the quinoa under cold water until water runs clear. In a saucepan, bring 1 cup of water to a boil. Add quinoa, reduce heat to low, cover, and simmer for 15 minutes or until water is absorbed. Remove from heat and let stand covered for 5 minutes. Fluff with a fork before serving.
2. While quinoa is cooking, heat a grill pan over medium-high heat. Rub the steak with half the olive oil, garlic, salt, and pepper. Place steak on the grill pan, cooking for about 4-5 minutes per

side for medium-rare, or until desired doneness. Remove from heat and let rest for a few minutes before slicing.

3. In a skillet over medium heat, add the remaining olive oil. Add green beans and season with salt and pepper. Cook, stirring occasionally, until beans are tender but still crisp, about 4-6 minutes.

4. Slice the steak into thin strips. Serve the grilled steak atop a bed of quinoa with green beans on the side. Garnish with fresh herbs.

Nutritional Information:

- Calories: 450
- Protein: 35g
- Carbohydrates: 33g
- Fiber: 6g
- Fat: 18g

Serving Size:

This recipe serves one, making it easy to manage portions and ensure you're eating just the right amount for weight loss and hormonal balance.

Cooking Time:

Preparation time is about 10 minutes, with a cooking time of approximately 20 minutes, totaling 30 minutes from start to finish.

Spaghetti Squash with Turkey Meatballs

Ingredients:

- 1 large spaghetti squash
- 1 pound ground turkey
- 1/2 cup finely chopped onion
- 2 cloves garlic, minced
- 1 egg, lightly beaten
- 1/4 cup grated Parmesan cheese
- 1/4 cup almond flour
- 2 tablespoons fresh parsley, chopped
- 1 teaspoon salt
- 1/2 teaspoon black pepper
- 1 cup marinara sauce, no sugar added
- 1 tablespoon olive oil

Instructions:

1. Preheat the oven to 400 degrees F (200 degrees C). Slice the spaghetti squash in half lengthwise and scoop out the seeds. Place the squash halves cut-side down on a baking sheet and roast for 40

minutes, or until the flesh is tender and can be shredded with a fork.

2. While the squash is roasting, combine ground turkey, onion, garlic, egg, Parmesan, almond flour, parsley, salt, and pepper in a bowl. Mix well and form into 1-inch meatballs.

3. Heat olive oil in a skillet over medium heat. Add meatballs and cook, turning occasionally, until browned on all sides, about 10 minutes. Pour marinara sauce over meatballs, cover, and simmer for another 10 minutes, or until meatballs are cooked through.

4. Remove the spaghetti squash from the oven, let it cool slightly, and then use a fork to scrape the inside, creating the "spaghetti."

5. Serve the spaghetti squash on plates and top with turkey meatballs and sauce.

Nutritional Information:

Each serving contains approximately:
- Calories: 320
- Protein: 22 g
- Fat: 18 g (Saturated: 4 g)
- Carbohydrates: 18 g (Fiber: 4 g, Sugars: 8 g)
- Sodium: 470 mg

Serving Size:

This recipe serves 4, with each serving consisting of approximately 1 cup of cooked spaghetti squash and 3-4 meatballs with sauce.

Cooking Time:

Total preparation and cooking time is approximately 60 minutes, which includes 40 minutes for roasting the squash and 20 minutes for preparing and cooking the meatballs.

Baked Cod with Lemon and Asparagus

Ingredients:

- 4 cod fillets (about 6 ounces each)
- 1 bunch of asparagus, trimmed
- 2 lemons, one sliced and one juiced
- 2 tablespoons of olive oil
- Salt and freshly ground black pepper, to taste
- Fresh parsley, chopped (for garnish)

Instructions:

1. Preheat your oven to 400 degrees Fahrenheit.
2. Arrange the asparagus in a single layer on a baking sheet, and drizzle with one tablespoon of olive oil, sprinkle with salt and pepper.
3. Place the cod fillets on top of the asparagus. Drizzle the fillets with the remaining olive oil and lemon juice. Season with salt and pepper, and top each fillet with a couple of lemon slices.
4. Bake in the preheated oven for about 12-15 minutes, or until the cod is opaque and flakes easily with a fork.
5. Remove from the oven and garnish with fresh parsley before serving.

Nutritional Information:

Each serving of this dish offers a balanced blend of nutrients, ideal for a PCOS diet:

- Calories: 200
- Carbohydrates: 5g
- Protein: 23g
- Fat: 10g
- Fiber: 2g

Serving Size:

This recipe serves four, with each serving consisting of one cod fillet and a quarter of the asparagus bunch.

Cooking Time:

The total preparation and cooking time is approximately 20 minutes, making this an excellent option for a quick and healthy lunch.

Stuffed Portobello Mushrooms with Spinach and Cheese

Ingredients:

- 4 large portobello mushroom caps, stems removed
- 1 tablespoon olive oil
- 2 cloves garlic, minced
- 4 cups fresh spinach
- 1/2 cup ricotta cheese
- 1/4 cup grated Parmesan cheese
- 1/4 teaspoon salt
- 1/4 teaspoon black pepper
- 1/4 cup shredded mozzarella cheese

Instructions:

1. Preheat the oven to 375 degrees Fahrenheit.
2. Brush the portobello mushrooms with olive oil and place them gill-side up on a baking sheet.
3. In a skillet over medium heat, sauté garlic in a splash of olive oil until fragrant, about 1 minute.
4. Add the spinach to the skillet and cook until wilted, about 3-4 minutes.

5. In a bowl, mix the wilted spinach, ricotta, Parmesan, salt, and pepper.
6. Divide the spinach and cheese mixture evenly among the mushroom caps, spooning it into the gill sides.
7. Top each mushroom with mozzarella cheese.
8. Bake in the preheated oven until the mushrooms are tender and the cheese is bubbly and golden, about 20 minutes.

Nutritional Information:

- Calories: 200
- Carbohydrates: 6 grams
- Protein: 12 grams
- Fat: 14 grams
- Fiber: 2 grams

Serving Size:

This recipe serves 4, with each serving consisting of one stuffed mushroom cap. This portion size is ideal for a satisfying lunch that won't spike blood sugar levels, supporting both weight loss and hormonal balance.

Cooking Time:

The total time required from start to finish is approximately 35 minutes, with 15 minutes of preparation and 20 minutes of cooking. This makes it a feasible option for a weekday lunch or a meal prep solution, ensuring that those on a tight schedule can still enjoy a nutritious, homemade meal.

Beef and Veggie Skewers with Brown Rice

Ingredients:

- 1 lb of lean beef, cut into 1-inch cubes
- 2 bell peppers (one red, one yellow), deseeded and cut into 1-inch pieces
- 1 large zucchini, sliced into half-inch rounds
- 1 large red onion, cut into chunks
- 2 tablespoons of olive oil
- 2 cloves garlic, minced
- 1 teaspoon of dried oregano
- 1 teaspoon of paprika
- Salt and pepper to taste
- 1 cup of brown rice

Instructions:

1. Begin by preparing the brown rice according to package instructions.
2. In a bowl, combine olive oil, garlic, oregano, paprika, salt, and pepper. Add the beef cubes to the marinade and let sit for at least 30 minutes in the refrigerator.

3. Preheat the grill to medium-high heat.
4. Thread the marinated beef, bell peppers, zucchini, and red onion onto skewers, alternating between the beef and vegetables.
5. Place the skewers on the grill and cook for about 10-12 minutes, turning occasionally, until the beef is cooked to your desired doneness and the vegetables are tender and slightly charred.
6. Serve the skewers over a bed of brown rice.

Nutritional Information:

Each serving of this meal provides approximately:
- Calories: 450
- Protein: 35g
- Carbohydrates: 45g (with 6g of dietary fiber)
- Fats: 15g (primarily from olive oil, which is rich in monounsaturated fats)

Serving Size:

The recipe serves four, with each serving including two skewers and a 3/4 cup of cooked brown rice.

Cooking Time:

- Prep time: 40 minutes (including marinating time)
- Cook time: 12 minutes

Eggplant Lasagna with Ricotta and Spinach

Ingredients:

- 2 large eggplants, sliced lengthwise into 1/4 inch thick strips
- 1 tablespoon olive oil
- 1 cup ricotta cheese
- 2 cups fresh spinach, chopped
- 1/2 cup grated Parmesan cheese
- 1 egg, beaten
- 2 cups marinara sauce, no sugar added
- 1 cup shredded mozzarella cheese
- Salt and pepper to taste
- Fresh basil for garnish

Instructions:

1. Preheat your oven to 375°F (190°C). Brush both sides of the eggplant slices with olive oil and season with salt and pepper. Arrange on a baking sheet in a single layer and roast in the oven for 15-20 minutes, turning once until the slices are just tender and lightly browned.

2. While the eggplant is roasting, mix ricotta cheese, spinach, Parmesan cheese, and the beaten egg in a bowl. Season with salt and pepper to taste.

3. Spread a thin layer of marinara sauce at the bottom of a baking dish. Layer the roasted eggplant slices over the sauce, then spread a portion of the ricotta mixture over the eggplant. Repeat the layers until all ingredients are used, finishing with a layer of marinara sauce. Top with shredded mozzarella cheese.

4. Bake in the preheated oven for 25-30 minutes or until the cheese is bubbly and golden brown.

5. Let the lasagna sit for 5-10 minutes before slicing. Garnish with fresh basil before serving.

Nutritional Information (per serving):

- Calories: 325
- Fat: 19g
- Carbohydrates: 22g
- Fiber: 6g
- Protein: 18g

Serving Size:

- This recipe yields six servings.

Cooking Time:

- Preparation time: 20 minutes
- Cooking time: 45-50 minutes
- Total time: About 1 hour and 10 minutes

Herb-Crusted Pork Tenderloin with Roasted Vegetables

Ingredients:

- 1 pork tenderloin (approximately 1-1.5 pounds)
- 2 tablespoons olive oil
- 1 tablespoon dried rosemary
- 1 tablespoon dried thyme
- 2 cloves garlic, minced
- Salt and pepper to taste
- 1 zucchini, sliced
- 1 red bell pepper, cut into 1-inch pieces
- 1 yellow bell pepper, cut into 1-inch pieces
- 2 medium carrots, sliced
- 1 tablespoon balsamic vinegar

Instructions:

1. Preheat your oven to 375°F (190°C).
2. In a small bowl, mix the olive oil, rosemary, thyme, garlic, salt, and pepper. Rub this mixture all over the pork tenderloin.
3. Place the tenderloin in the center of a large baking dish. Surround it with the sliced zucchini, bell peppers, and carrots.

4. Drizzle the vegetables with balsamic vinegar and a bit more olive oil, tossing them to coat.

5. Roast in the preheated oven for 25-30 minutes, or until the pork reaches an internal temperature of 145°F (63°C) and the vegetables are tender and caramelized.

6. Remove from oven and let the pork rest for 5 minutes before slicing. Serve warm.

Nutritional Information:

Each serving (1 slice of pork with a serving of vegetables) contains approximately:
- Calories: 220
- Protein: 24g
- Fat: 10g (of which 2g is saturated)
- Carbohydrates: 8g
- Fiber: 2g
- Sugar: 3g

Serving Size:

This recipe serves 4 people. Each serving consists of about 3-4 slices of pork and a generous helping of roasted vegetables.

Cooking Time:

Total preparation and cooking time is approximately 35-40 minutes, making it an efficient option for a nourishing and fulfilling lunch.

Chickpea Curry with Brown Rice and Spinach

Ingredients:

- 1 tablespoon olive oil
- 1 large onion, finely chopped
- 2 cloves garlic, minced
- 1 tablespoon grated ginger
- 1 tablespoon curry powder
- 1 teaspoon ground cumin
- 1 teaspoon turmeric
- 1 can (15 ounces) chickpeas, rinsed and drained
- 1 can (14 ounces) diced tomatoes, with juice
- 1 can (14 ounces) coconut milk
- 4 cups fresh spinach leaves
- Salt and pepper, to taste
- 2 cups cooked brown rice

Instructions:

1. Heat the olive oil in a large skillet over medium heat. Add the onion, garlic, and ginger, sautéing until the onion becomes translucent.

2. Stir in the curry powder, cumin, and turmeric, cooking for about 1 minute until fragrant.
3. Add the chickpeas, tomatoes with their juice, and coconut milk. Bring the mixture to a boil, then reduce the heat and simmer for 15 minutes.
4. Stir in the spinach and continue to cook until the spinach wilts, about 3 minutes. Season with salt and pepper to taste.
5. Serve the curry over cooked brown rice.

Nutritional Information:

- Calories: 345 per serving
- Protein: 9 grams
- Fat: 17 grams (saturated fat: 7 grams)
- Carbohydrates: 42 grams
- Fiber: 8 grams
- Sugar: 5 grams

Serving Size:

- This recipe yields 4 servings.

Cooking Time:

- Prep time: 10 minutes
- Cook time: 25 minutes
- Total time: 35 minutes

Chapter 4: Snacks and Desserts

Dark Chocolate and Almond Energy Bites

Ingredients:

- 1 cup rolled oats
- 1/2 cup almond butter
- 1/4 cup ground flaxseed
- 1/4 cup honey or agave syrup (for a vegan option)
- 1/2 cup dark chocolate chips (at least 70% cocoa)
- 1/3 cup chopped almonds
- 1 teaspoon vanilla extract

Instructions:

1. In a large bowl, mix the oats, almond butter, ground flaxseed, honey, and vanilla extract until well combined.
2. Fold in the dark chocolate chips and chopped almonds.
3. Refrigerate the mixture for about 30 minutes until it's firm enough to shape.
4. Roll the mixture into balls of about one inch in diameter.
5. Place the energy bites on a baking sheet lined with parchment paper and refrigerate again for an hour or until firm.

Nutritional Information:

Each energy bite contains approximately:
- Calories: 150
- Protein: 4 grams
- Fat: 9 grams (with only 2 grams of saturated fat from the dark chocolate)
- Carbohydrates: 15 grams
- Fiber: 3 grams

Serving Size:

This recipe makes about 15 energy bites. A serving size is typically 1-2 energy bites, making it an ideal snack size for mid-morning or afternoon.

Cooking Time:

Preparation time is about 15 minutes, with an additional waiting time of 1.5 hours for the mixture to firm up.

Greek Yogurt Parfait with Honey and Nuts

Ingredients:

- 1 cup plain Greek yogurt
- 2 tablespoons raw honey
- 1/4 cup mixed nuts (almonds, walnuts, and pecans), roughly chopped
- 1/2 teaspoon vanilla extract
- A pinch of cinnamon (optional)

Instructions:

1. In a serving bowl or glass, layer half of the Greek yogurt.
2. Drizzle one tablespoon of honey over the yogurt.
3. Add half of the chopped nuts over the honey.
4. Repeat the layering with the remaining yogurt, honey, and nuts.
5. Top with a sprinkle of cinnamon and vanilla extract for added flavor.
6. Serve immediately or refrigerate for up to an hour before serving to allow the flavors to meld.

Nutritional Information:

This parfait is not only a delight to the taste buds but also offers substantial nutritional benefits. Each serving provides approximately:
- Calories: 310
- Protein: 20 grams
- Carbohydrates: 26 grams (from honey and a small amount from nuts)
- Fats: 15 grams (primarily healthy fats from nuts)
- Fiber: 3 grams
- This snack is rich in protein from the Greek yogurt, which can aid in muscle repair and satiety. The nuts add a healthy dose of fats and fiber, which are crucial for hormonal balance and sustained energy levels.

Serving Size:

The above ingredients make for one serving, ideal for one person as a filling snack or a dessert alternative.

Cooking Time:

The Greek Yogurt Parfait with Honey and Nuts requires no actual cooking, making it a quick and easy option. The preparation time is roughly 5 minutes, which involves merely assembling the ingredients.

Chia Seed Pudding with Mango

Ingredients:

- 1/4 cup chia seeds
- 1 cup unsweetened almond milk
- 1 tablespoon honey or a preferred natural sweetener
- 1/2 teaspoon vanilla extract
- 1 ripe mango, peeled and diced
- A pinch of salt

Instructions:

1. In a mixing bowl, combine chia seeds, almond milk, honey, vanilla extract, and a pinch of salt. Stir well to evenly distribute the chia seeds.
2. Cover the bowl and refrigerate for at least 4 hours, preferably overnight, allowing the chia seeds to swell and absorb the liquid, forming a pudding-like consistency.
3. Once set, stir the pudding to check consistency. If it's too thick, add a bit more almond milk until the desired consistency is achieved.
4. Serve the pudding in individual bowls or glasses and top with freshly diced mango.

Nutritional Information:

Each serving of Chia Seed Pudding with Mango offers a balanced mix of nutrients conducive to managing PCOS symptoms. It contains approximately:

- Calories: 215
- Protein: 4 grams
- Carbohydrates: 35 grams
- Fats: 7 grams
- Fiber: 10 grams

Serving Size:

The recipe serves 2. It can be doubled or halved to accommodate more or fewer servings depending on personal or family needs.

Cooking Time:

The active preparation time for this recipe is around 10 minutes, with an additional 4 hours or overnight for the pudding to set properly in the refrigerator.

Apple Slices with Almond Butter

Ingredients:
- 1 medium apple, cored and sliced
- 2 tablespoons of almond butter

Instructions:
1. Core and slice the apple into thin pieces.
2. Spread almond butter evenly over each apple slice.

Nutritional Information:
- Calories: 280
- Carbohydrates: 34g
- Protein: 4g
- Fat: 16g
- Fiber: 6g

Serving Size:
- This recipe serves 1, making it a perfect, quick snack for any time of the day.

Cooking Time:

- Prep time: 5 minutes
- Cook time: 0 minutes

Roasted Chickpeas with Spices

Ingredients:

- 1 can (15 oz) chickpeas, drained and rinsed
- 1 tablespoon olive oil
- 1/2 teaspoon smoked paprika
- 1/2 teaspoon ground cumin
- 1/4 teaspoon garlic powder
- 1/4 teaspoon onion powder
- 1/4 teaspoon salt
- 1/8 teaspoon cayenne pepper (optional)

Instructions:

1. Preheat your oven to 400 degrees Fahrenheit (200 degrees Celsius).
2. Pat the chickpeas dry with paper towels, removing as much moisture as possible.
3. In a bowl, toss the chickpeas with olive oil and all the spices until evenly coated.
4. Spread the chickpeas on a baking sheet in a single layer.
5. Roast in the preheated oven for 20-30 minutes, or until crisp and golden. Shake the pan or stir the chickpeas halfway through to ensure even cooking.

6. Remove from the oven and let cool on the baking sheet to enhance their crunchiness.

Nutritional Information (per serving):

- Calories: 134
- Protein: 4g
- Fat: 5g
- Carbohydrates: 18g
- Fiber: 5g
- Sugar: 0g

Serving Size:

- Makes 4 servings, approximately 1/4 cup per serving

Cooking Time:

- Preparation time: 5 minutes
- Cooking time: 20-30 minutes

Conclusion

As we reach the conclusion of the PCOS Diet Cookbook for Weight Loss, it's clear that managing PCOS through diet is not only possible but also empowering and enjoyable. This cookbook is designed to be a comprehensive resource, providing more than just recipes; it offers a holistic approach to managing PCOS symptoms and achieving weight loss goals.

The carefully curated recipes focus on balancing hormones, improving insulin sensitivity, and reducing inflammation, all of which are critical for managing PCOS. By integrating whole foods, lean proteins, healthy fats, and fiber-rich ingredients into your meals, you can create a sustainable eating pattern that supports your health and well-being.

The cookbook also emphasizes the importance of practicality and adaptability. With easy-to-follow recipes that fit into a busy lifestyle, meal planning templates, and modifications for various dietary restrictions, it ensures that everyone can benefit from its guidance. The aim is to make healthy eating accessible and enjoyable, removing the stress and guesswork from meal preparation.

Beyond the recipes, this cookbook advocates for a holistic lifestyle approach. Stress management techniques, regular physical activity, and consistent sleep schedules are highlighted as vital components of managing PCOS effectively. These lifestyle changes, combined with a balanced diet, can lead to significant improvements in your overall health, energy levels, and quality of life.

One of the most valuable aspects of this cookbook is the sense of community it fosters. By encouraging readers to share their experiences, challenges, and successes, it builds a supportive network of individuals who understand the unique struggles of living with PCOS. This community aspect can provide motivation and encouragement, making the journey to better health feel less isolating.

As you implement the strategies and recipes from this cookbook, remember that consistency is key. The changes might be gradual, but with persistence, you will start to notice positive shifts in your health and well-being. Celebrate these small victories and stay committed to your goals, knowing that every step you take is a step towards a healthier, more balanced life.

In conclusion, the PCOS Diet Cookbook for Weight Loss is more than just a collection of recipes; it is a guide to transforming your relationship with food and your body. By understanding the impact of diet on PCOS and making informed, nutritious choices, you can manage your symptoms effectively and achieve your weight loss goals. Embrace this journey with an open heart and a determined spirit, and let this cookbook be your trusted companion on the path to health and wellness.

www.ingramcontent.com/pod-product-compliance
Lightning Source LLC
Chambersburg PA
CBHW071941210526
45479CB00002B/766